How to Effectively Use Honey as Medicine
What Doctors Don't Tell You

Transform Your Health with Nature's Living Food

Ruth Tan

Eating for health has never been sweeter.

How to Effectively Use Honey as Medicine: What Doctors Don't Tell You

All Copyright 2010.

All rights reserved. No part of this publication may be reproduced, stored in a retrieval system, or transmitted in any form or by any means, electronics, mechanical, photocopying, recording or otherwise, without the prior permission of the publication.

Note to the Reader

All pages and contents presented are intended for informational and educational purposes and should not be construed as professional medical diagnoses, advice or instruction, which can only be given by your personal health care provider. This book does not officially endorse the use of alternative therapies over conventional medicine. You should never disregard medical advice or delay in seeking it because of something you have read here. The author shall have neither liability nor responsibility to any person or entity with respect to any loss, damage, or injury caused or alleged to be caused directly or indirectly by the information contained in this book.

What's In It?

Contents

Fact or Fiction?..6

Preface 7

Sweet and Sticky Truth?..................................12

What's in Honey?..13

Honey and Table Sugar Aren't Equal 15

Honey as Home Remedy.................................17

Miracle Cure for Sore Throats and Coughs 19

Natural Sweetener for Good Health 21

Honey Lemon Weight Loss Tip......................27

Drink Honey Vinegar to Health 29

Honey Cinnamon Fights Obesity and Many Other Health Problems 33

Restoring Health & Losing Weight with The Hibernation Diet..37

Honey is Anti-Cancer.....................................42

My First Honey Water Fast 44

Nature's First Aid Burn Treatment................52

Honey Skin Care 54

More Health Benefits of Honey 59

The Honey Allergy Debate 61

I'm Diabetic, Can I Eat Honey?.......................................64

Why Babies Should Not Be Given Honey?....................66

Are all Honey Varieties Equal?.....................................68

UMF Manuka Honey 70

Forms and Types of Honey 73

What is "Pure Honey"? 77

How Much Honey is Excessive? 79

How to Best Store Honey?..81

Honey in Singapore...84

Easy "Ready-to-Go" Honey Recipes.............................87

30 Questions with Answers 92

About the Author 105

Fact or Fiction?

1. Honey is sweeter than table sugar.
2. Honey is best taken when mixed in hot water.
3. Honey never spoils, even when it's stored open.
4. Honey comes in the liquid, cream, and powder form.
5. Honey's quality is not affected by crystallisation.
6. Honey contains no cholesterol.
7. Honey contains only a tiny amount of fat.
8. Honey helps burn fats when we sleep.
9. Honey labelled as "raw" is not heated at all.
10. Honey is suitable for people of any age.
11. Honey should not be ingested by pregnant women.
12. Honey is harmful for diabetics.

Before you leaf through the pages, test yourself how much you know about honey with the above statements. By the time you arrive at the last page of this book, you would have derived all the answers – whether each of the above 12 statements is a "fact" or "fiction".

Enjoy!

Preface

Healthy are those who eat honey.

Each time someone found out I was running a website on honey, he or she would surely query if I owned a honey shop. And when they learnt I didn't, it became puzzling to them why I would choose "honey" over all the web topics in this world. Could I be any more boring? It is "uncool" to be associated with an old-fashioned food like honey. Only old folks, grannies, and honey farmers are keen on eating and discussing honey, so they say. Do they know what honey is? Yes, they do - It's a sweet liquid made by the bees, and period.

I agree that topics like the crazy Botox mania, promising Acai Berry juice, hottest slimming diet fad, latest spa experience, most acclaimed anti-aging supplements, or the big yoga craze would probably be more appealing to the modern crowd. Yes, I could have pursued the latest health buzz instead. But everyone has a story to tell, and so do I.

My love for honey is an ironical one. Born and bred in the city, I never knew what it was like to live in a farm and was never close to Mother Nature. In fact, nature, whether it was to do with the flowers, shrubs, herbs, vegetation, trees, bees, birds, animals or any living thing or creature or of any kind, had been remote in my growing up years. They were at best objects that appeared only in schools, books and media or existed in figments of my imagination. Closer to my heart were the electronics, media, digital gadgets, and communication devices. (Yes, you are right, I was deprived. And in fact, I'm terribly afraid of creepy crawlies, including bees. It's a psychological, irrational fear of hearing the buzz...)

It was the year 2006 when I chanced upon the different varieties of honey in the shops. My sweet tooth was responsible for loving almost anything sweet. The vast differences in the tastes and even prices of honey types intrigued me. The more I researched on honey and consulted the experts about it, the more wowed I was. And when studies turned up more and more evidence of the medical benefits of honey, to be truthful, I was both fascinated and sceptical at the same time. How can something so sweet possibly be of any benefit to health? My disbelief spurred me to find out even more, setting me wonderfully on the road of discovering and experimenting with honey.

The amazing thing is, ever since I started the habit of taking two tablespoons of honey before bedtime, I found that my body constitution improved gradually and steadily. This led to reduced doctor visits and missed work days. From time to time, I still had bouts of sore-throats, but they were mild and over in a day or two.

You probably need to know how weak I was before. My childhood was littered with frequent bouts of fever, serious sore throat and chronic coughs. While the Chinese physicians claimed I had a weak body constitution and my "Yin and Yang" energies were said to be out of balance, the Western doctors diagnosed that I had tonsillitis and naturally extra-sensitive airways. I was frequently troubled by throat inflammations. Each sore throat episode repeatedly led to a vicious cycle of fever, followed by a prolonged, debilitating cough which would take weeks or even sometimes a couple of months to recover after a few visits to the doctor. The Chinese called it "100-day cough". From the age of fourteen to sixteen, wherever I went, I had to carry a blue puffer (quick-relief inhaler) prescribed by the throat, ear, and nose specialist. It seemed that as I grew up, I gradually got out of this the asthmatic cough, but still, I had to visit the doctor about ten times or more a year. (In case you are not too familiar with my country, Singapore, people don't practice much of self-medication here. We go to the commonly available and accessible clinics and let the doctors diagnose and dispense us the medicine prescribed. Some people don't even take note of the names of the medicine given by the doctors in the clinics. Self-care is not too popular an idea here.)

For many years after delivering my first daughter, I wrestled with syndromes of adrenal fatigue. Especially in the evening after a day's work, I would feel totally frazzled and washed out like a sick parrot, as if all my bones were falling apart and every bit of energy had been drained out. Turning in early and waking up late didn't work; sleep just could not relieve me of the frequent, intense exhaustion. After what seemed like an eternity of putting up with that run-down feeling, I eventually learned how to consistently incorporate honey into my diet over time. Gradually, honey not only propped me up with positive energy and sustained me throughout the day, but also supplied me a special dose of energy to exercise. Barely capable of jogging for a straight ten-minute, I was probably the world's worst jogger. And I often felt embarrassed by my own jogging pace that was apparently slower than people who were strolling. After taking honey for several weeks, for the first time in my life I felt bounce in my steps. I didn't become an athlete but at least managing a 1.5km jog for about three to four times a week turned out to be an easy feat me. I was so enthused to have discovered and experienced the first health benefit of honey – its anabolic ability.

Another significant change that steadily came along was my sleep quality. For the longest time, I had to wake up to go to the bathroom about two, three times at night. Attributing it to an irritable bladder, I had never seen any doctor for it. Now with the consistent daily consumption of honey before bedtime, getting up at night has been reduced to once or none. I believe this is just going to get better.

The three-day honey fast had proven beneficial in terms of body detoxification. It did take a tremendous lot of determination to stop eating and not think about food for three to five days, but eating honey as part of the fast had made the experience a lot easier and motivating. But what was most important was that this practice had helped to improve my bowel movements (from every two or three days a bowel movement to every day).

It is my hope that my fanaticism for honey and a compilation of my stories from my journey with honey would inspire others to make this statement, "I never knew this big deal about honey!" Surely, this golden liquid must be given a much more pronounced food status than what it's currently now. We need to see a brewing interest and curiosity in this natural sweetener and a growing number of people tapping on its amazing goodness. While so people are jumping on the latest diet fad, coveting the wonder anti-aging cream, and chasing after the newest health pill, I want to create some attention for this precious, age-old food, which I strongly believe can significantly better the health of this generation and the generations to come.

Eating for health has never been sweeter.

Sweet and Sticky Truth?

Who doesn't fancy sweet bites, everybody does.

But it is hard for sweet foods (especially very sweet ones) to earn credibility as a health food. And I find this particularly true with this caramel-like liquid, honey. People spontaneously associate sweet liquids with extra calories, weight gain, diabetes, tooth decay, hyperactivity, poor immune system, obesity, and a myriad of health and diet sabotages. It is probably a lot easier to convince someone to swallow bitter pills for health than to convert someone to eat honey for health. The old adage "no pain, no gain" works powerfully in the minds of people. Certainly I am able to grasp this mentality because I too was once sceptic as well.

So what is honey? Why is this golden liquid special? Isn't it made of sugars? How healthy can sugar be?

Read on, and you'll have the sweet secrets revealed, one by one.

"Oh the powers of nature. She knows what we need, and the doctors know nothing."

~Benvenuto Cellini

What's in Honey?

A source of carbohydrates, honey contains 80% natural sugar, mostly fructose and glucose, 18% water, and 2% minerals, vitamins, pollen and protein.

Nectar itself is composed mainly of sucrose and water. Bees add enzymes that create additional chemical compounds, inverting the sucrose into fructose and glucose, and then evaporate the water so that the resulting product will resist spoiling.

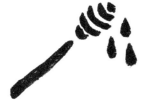

Due to the high level of fructose, this natural sweetener is sweeter than table sugar. The vitamins present in honey are B6, B1, B2 and B5. The minerals found in honey include calcium, copper, iron, magnesium, manganese, phosphorus, potassium, sodium and zinc. Honey also has antioxidants and amino acids, the building blocks of proteins. It's sodium-free, fat-free, and cholesterol-free!

One tablespoon of natural sweetener honey contains 64 calories, while one tablespoon of table sugar or sucrose contains 46 calories. Though honey may have more calories, we actually need to use less of it since it is sweeter than table sugar. As a result, you may in fact consume even less amount of calories that you would with sugar. Our taste buds can sometimes be deceived, and our diet sabotaged by the amount of sugar in the foods we eat. Would you be taken aback if I tell you how much table sugar is in a can of coke? 10 teaspoons! And a 50g chocolate bar? 7 teaspoons!

Honey and Table Sugar Aren't Equal

"Sugar is sugar, honey is made up of sugar and is not more healthful than table sugar, as far as our body is concerned, there is no difference between honey and table sugar." Correct?

Wrong. Indeed, both honey and white sugar are made up of fructose and glucose, but there is a big difference between natural sugar from honey and sugar from highly processed white sugar. It's the same when we compare fruits and honey, the sugars in both are also scientifically called fructose and glucose, however in reality, both are different types of sugar from different sources, with different health benefits and effects.

These are two key differences that clearly set honey apart from table sugar:

One:
Table sugar is sucrose, which is made up of two molecules bonded together. When we eat table sugar, our stomach has to use its own enzymes to separate the molecules apart before we can use the sugar's energy. Honey is quite different. The bees have added a special enzyme to the nectar that divides the sucrose into glucose and fructose -- two simple sugars that our bodies can absorb directly.

Hence, compared to table sugar, honey has a healthier Glycemic Index (GI) which measures the negative impact of a given food on the blood-glucose level. Honey's Glycemic Index is 55, while sucrose's Glycemic

Index, 61.The lower the GI rating, the slower the absorption and infusion of sugars into the bloodstream and hence a more gradual and healthier digestion process.

Two:
Unlike honey, table sugar lacks minerals and vitamins (hence the latter often has been called empty calories) and draws upon the body's nutrients to be metabolized into the system. When these nutrients are all used up, metabolizing of undesirable cholesterol and fatty acid is impeded, contributing to higher cholesterol and promoting obesity as a result of the accumulated fatty acid on the organs and tissues. That is why it is not uncommon for fat people to suffer from malnutrition and many other health related problems. Hence, whether your idea is to work towards a healthier body or a more ideal waistline, honey will be a smarter choice than table sugar.

Besides the differences in nutrition, table sugar can never compete with honey in taste. Though both are sweet, the range of honey floral varieties is so vast that experiencing the uniqueness of each variety and being able to appropriate each variety and exploit every possibility to complement and improve taste of different types of foods becomes a skilful art.

Honey as Home Remedy

I am sure many of us have at some point or another sought, heard, or read about the use of natural medicine in Ayurveda and Traditional Chinese Medicine but had never really understood the cause and effect in those remedies. And doctors often keep mum about the effectiveness of those home cures ranted and raved by our grandparents. Nevertheless, despite all the criticism, time-honoured home remedies continue to have its remarkable appeal in the arena of healing.

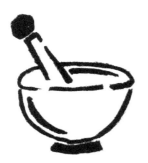

Many of these natural cures are often seen as a more effective and holistic form of therapy for health conditions that are not exactly so critically emergent and do not require an immediate treatment but yet can be so chronic that it takes a toll on the body over the long run if not properly attended to. Yes, alternative medicine is gaining popularity in this modern age despite the ever increasing haste in introducing advanced technologies and synthetic drugs for diseases and ailments.

Honey home remedies existed even before the advent of modern medicine and have been tried and tested by diverse cultures and peoples from all over the world. Even with the lack of endorsement of medical doctors and scientific basis of belief and trust, honey has continued to thrive as alternative medicine for a plethora of ailments such as cough, sore throat, obesity, burns, dull skin, sleeplessness, and yeast infection, all of which I'll share with you the relevance of honey as a medicine.

Miracle Cure for Sore Throats and Coughs

I shall kick off with honey's most well-known benefit -- its effectiveness as a natural lozenge and a cough syrup. Thanks to its antimicrobial properties, honey not only soothes throat but can also kill certain bacteria causing the infection!

Professional singers commonly use honey to soothe their throat before performances. And the Chinese believe that excess "heatiness" in the body causes throat inflammation and taking honey drink can be helpful. Direction for application: Gargle with a mixture of two tablespoons of honey, four tablespoons of lemon juice and a pinch of salt.

Many scientists believe that honey, a traditional, natural home remedy for cough can offer a "safe and legitimate alternative" to Dextromethorphan (DM), which can occasionally causes severe side-effects in children, including muscle contractions and spasms due to the strong chemical make-up. A study (2007) by researchers from Penn State College of Medicine, US, involved 105 children with coughs between the ages of 2 and 18. Before bed, the children were given artificial honey-flavoured DM cough syrup, buckwheat honey or nothing at all. Results revealed that parents of children who received the honey rated their children's sleep and symptoms as better! It was believed that honey's ability as a home remedy for cough may be due to the way it soothes on contact and stimulates saliva.

The following is a testimony that I received from an Indian web visitor who had seen how honey had worked powerfully for coughs:

"My servant was having cough for almost a month, we had taken him to doctor who prescribed him very high antibiotics, which had to be taken for four days. Since there was no improvement, somebody suggested searching in internet for home remedies. There I read that if honey mixed with black pepper is taken two to three times a day, cough will go. Surprisingly we started giving him honey mixed with black pepper and his cough was cured completely in five days."

While many have reported mixing honey with lemon grass juice, cayenne pepper, ground ginger, or garlic and taking two to three times a day to be beneficial in treating cough, I have personally found taking raw honey directly to be very effective for cough and sore throats. Simply scoop a tablespoon of raw honey, leave it in the mouth and coat the throat for as long as possible until all is dissolved and swallowed. This will almost immediately ease the pain of the strep throat, reduce phlegm and relieve cough. (Note: Honey varieties that are candy-thick work perfectly well.)

Next time, if you or someone in your family had a cough, remember honey as a natural alternative medicine.

Natural Sweetener for Good Health
Watch out for Dangerous Sweeteners!

As we know, sugars are one form of carbohydrates essential for our body's energy supply. However, excessive sugar consumption is a major contributor to calorie intake and weight gain. It can also deplete your body of several minerals and vitamins, such as Vitamin C.

Nutritionists consider Vitamin C to be the single most important supplemental nutrient for the proper functioning of white blood cells and maintaining a strong, efficient immune system and recovering from infections. The white blood cells in our body need high doses of Vitamin C to fight viruses and bacteria, and combat illnesses such as the common cold, heart disease, cancer and osteoporosis. Glucose and Vitamin C have similar chemical structures, thus when the sugar levels go up, they compete for one another when entering the cells. Hence, as you eat more sugar, there will be more glucose around and less Vitamin C will be allowed into the cell, resulting the slowing down of your immune system.

Simple sugars found in foods that do not use a natural sweetener have been observed to aggravate illness such as asthma, hypertension, arthritis, nervous disorders, diabetes, heart diseases, gallstones, and mood swings. They are certainly not a preferred form of carbohydrates in our meals. If you are one of those parents who would try to keep all the candies and sweets away from their young children whenever they are down with flu and cough but do not know exactly the logic of it, now you understand it!

Different types of carbohydrates behave differently in the body and are part of different nutritional packages. Over-processed, factory-made sugars or table sugar, and even raw or brown sugar which do not have any vitamins or whatsoever nutrients may not be the best choice of carbohydrates. In fact, they are foes of the healthy immune system – they suppress immune cells. For instance, a chocolate bar may satisfy hunger because of the high amount of sugar and fat, but it can create a nutrient deficit in the body. That explains why there are so many overweight people who are at the same time under-nourished and in poor health!

Nonetheless, trying to fight sweet tooth by eliminating sugar from your meals may not be the smartest choice. We tend to crave for even more sweet foods and end up with more dreadful binge eating. If you are watching your waistline, consider replacing man-made, processed, empty calories in your diet with honey, a natural sweetener.

The best types of food not only provide a steady supply of energy but also bring other nutrients the body needs. While refined dietary sugars lack minerals and vitamins, honey contains the extra nutrition of amino acids and a variety of minerals essential for its metabolism. Try raw honey spread on a slice of bread. The plant enzyme amylase present in the raw honey is effective in breaking down and helping the pre-digestion of the starches in the bread. Taking honey also helps to raise the level of antioxidants required in the body.

Artificial Sweetener: Aspartame

In our constant battle of the bulge, we often turn to low-calorie foods and artificial sweeteners like Aspartame in hope of satisfying those sweet cravings without the added calories. The bad news is you could be putting yourself completely on the wrong track. These chemical laden sweeteners might get you off from a few calories but it might also give you a bunch of other serious health problems.

Aspartame, commercially known as Equal and Nutrasweet, has a flavour similar to sucrose, and also acts as a taste intensifier and enhancer. It is 200 times sweeter than sucrose but has a "flat" taste -- I am sure many people who have a sweet tooth knows what I am talking about, that means it basically has no aftertaste. A sachet of this artificial sweetener is equivalent in sweetness to two teaspoons of sugar (32 calories), for just four calories, an amount which is insignificant.

In 1981, the FDA approved Aspartame and declared it to be safe for use in a variety of products, as a table-top sweetener and in carbonated beverages. In the recent years, you might have noticed that on the store shelves there are more and more variety of foods which claim "sugar free". In 1993, approval of Aspartame was made as well for use in hard and soft candies, baked goods and mixes, non-alcoholic beverages and malt beverages. However, there has been a lot of debate over the health concerns caused by this artificial sweetener which has been reported to be unsafe for humans. Serious reactions including seizures, nervous system damage and neurological troubles have been linked to this sugar substitute. With so much argument about its health hazards and until researchers turn in more scientific conclusions, this sweetener may not be the wisest diet product for those eagerly trying to lose weight and diabetics who are looking for table sugar substitutes to improve their health condition. Many studies have also supported the recommendation that pregnant women, nursing mothers, infants and children should avoid products containing the sweetener.

Refined Sugar: High Fructose Corn Syrup

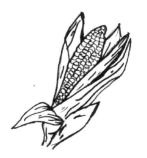

"Fructose" and "corn" conjure in our minds images of juicy corn ears and baskets of fresh fruits. The name high fructose corn syrup sounds rather harmless, and in fact even suggests substances that are natural and healthy, but what exactly is it?

High Fructose Corn Syrup is far from natural. White corn starch processed from genetically modified corns is made to yield glucose under high temperature. The glucose is then converted into fructose. Being a highly processed sweetener, HFCS is synthetic! A Study by Institute of Agriculture and Trade Policy (2009) even revealed that some of this syrup is manufactured using mercury-grade caustic soda. Mercury accumulates in the body, and is especially damaging to the developing brain of the foetus and infant. Pregnant moms, watch what you are drinking.

Refined HFCS is metabolized by your liver and does not cause the pancreas to release insulin the way the body normally does. Thus it converts to fat more than any other sugar. Kidney specialists at the University of Florida, discovered that fructose consumption raised blood levels of uric acid and developed "metabolic syndrome," a condition of insulin resistance and abdominal obesity linked to heart disease and diabetes. In 2009, a study conducted on rats by the University of Washington revealed that moderate consumption of fructose and high fructose corn syrup-sweetened beverages leads to significant degradation of the lipids in the liver. It also pointed to significant rises in both cholesterol and triglyceride levels in rats fed on fructose-sweetened beverages. A press release by the American Chemical Society also informed that researchers have found that commonly consumed carbonated beverages sweetened with HFCS had high levels of reactive compounds that have the potential to the development of diabetes, particularly in children. If all these findings do not stir us to fret about the health and future of our children, I don't know what will.

The sticky truth is that corn syrup has sneaked into so many foods, e.g. sauces, peanut butter, cereals, yoghurts, salad dressings, cookies, processed meats, etc, you just name it. Its low cost and long shelf-life have caused many food manufacturers to embrace it so much that you can only detect it with enough vigilance in your shopping. Furthermore, corn syrup easily results in overeating because it fails to stimulate leptin, the hormone that triggers chemical signals to tell the brain your stomach is full, like other foods containing regular refined sugar do. And, what is even more disturbing is, when HFCS is heated/cooked, it becomes contaminated with hydroxymethylfurfural (HMF). And when HMF breaks down in the human body, they become even more toxic than HMF itself. HFCS is banned in Europe and Canada for reasons.

Most people have been told that HFCS is bad, but they don't really know why. Get the facts right and help save our children from drowning in high fructose corn syrup, HFCS. No schools, educational institutions or religious organisations are going to educate them on agri-corporate hogwash and the harmful effects of HFCS.

Remember, the type of food you consume is very important for your health. "You are what you eat."

Honey Lemon Weight Loss Tip

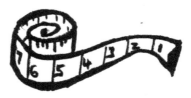

Obesity is the physical condition of the body when excessive deposition of fat takes place in the tissues, putting a strain on the heart, kidneys, liver and the joints such as the hips, knees and ankles and thus, overweight people are susceptible to several diseases like diabetes, high blood pressure, arthritis, liver, and gall bladder disorders.

The honey and lemon recipe is a one of the hottest favourites among honey enthusiasts who are seeking out ways to shed the pounds without the loss of energy and appetite, because making it just can't get any easier.

It is believed that drinking lemon juice, an alkaline food, with a little honey the first thing in the morning is an effective anti-cellulite treatment as it helps to increase body metabolism by mobilizing the extra deposited fat in the body allowing it to be utilized as energy for normal functions. If you are determined to shed weight and speed up your sluggish metabolism, try this honey and lemon diet tip.

It is easy to prepare this natural cure: Mix one teaspoon of raw honey (unheated) with the juice of two teaspoons of lime or lemon juice in a glass of room temperature or lukewarm water (not boiling water!). Take this remedy once in the morning on an empty stomach. It is commonly said that this simple delicious drink taken after a big and oily meal, is an effective digestive and detoxification tonic.

Drink Honey Vinegar to Health

The apple cider vinegar and honey drink has traditionally been used as an at-home self remedy for many ailments, and even as an anti-aging elixir. Many people have recognised and made use of its cleansing and disinfecting properties to self-detoxify their body. It is seen as a powerful cleansing agent and natural medicine with naturally occurring antibiotic and antiseptic that fights germs and bacteria. The ailments that could be cured by this apple cider vinegar and honey treatment include premature aging, obesity, heat exhaustion, heartburn, bad breath, arthritis, high blood pressure, and high cholesterol level.

In 1958, D.C. Jarvis, M.D. published the book titled Folk Medicine: A Vermont Doctor's Guide to Good Health, recommending apple cider vinegar as a powerful alternative medicine. His advice was that mixing the apple cider vinegar with honey enhanced the healing power of the vinegar. Jarvis also wrote that apple cider vinegar could destroy harmful bacteria in the digestive tract and suggested it as a digestive tonic to be consumed with meals. Folk Medicine became a bestseller a year later. According to Time magazine, it sold hundreds of thousands copies in a single week and received many testimonials by people who had benefited from the apple cider vinegar and honey mixture.

How does this vinegar and honey remedy actually work? A person's bloodstream tends toward becoming acidic with our modern diet of fats, starches and processed foods, e.g. fast foods, meats, peanuts, seafood, alcohol and coffee. If your body is acidic, disease can flourish; and if it is alkaline, it is in balance and can fight off germs and ailments such as bladder and kidney conditions, osteoporosis, brittle bones, joint pains, aching muscles, low energy and chronic fatigue, and slow digestion.

Raw fruits, leafy green vegetables, legumes, and tea are examples of alkaline forming foods. Interestingly and ironically, a food's acid or alkaline-forming tendency in the body has nothing to do with the actual pH of the food itself. For instance, lemons and limes are very acidic; however the end-products they produce after digestion and assimilation are very alkaline so lemons and limes are alkaline-forming in the body. Likewise, meat will test alkaline before digestion but it leaves very acidic residue in the body so, like nearly all animal products, meat is acid-forming.

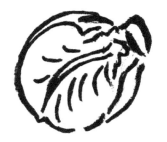

It is important to know that stomach acid or the pH of the stomach is an entirely different matter from the pH of the body's fluids and tissues. The body has an acid-alkaline (or acid-base) ratio called the pH which is a balance between positively charges ions (acid-forming) and negatively charged ions (alkaline-forming). When this balance is compromised, many problems can occur.

The body is forced to borrow minerals—including calcium, sodium, potassium and magnesium from vital organs and bones to neutralize the acid and safely remove it from the body. And severe damage can be done to the body due to high acidity. Ideally, for most people, the ideal diet is 75 percent alkalizing and 25 percent acidifying foods by volume. Allergic reactions and other forms of stress also tend to produce excessive acids in the body.

The alkalinity of apple cider vinegar can correct excess acidity in our system and help prevent and fight infection. Honey enhances the healing properties of the vinegar, as well as improves the taste of the mixture. Essentially, to prepare:

1. Mix a tablespoon of apple cider vinegar and a tablespoon of raw honey.

   (Apple cider vinegar is actually made from fresh, organic, crushed apples that are allowed to mature naturally in wooden barrels, but you can get it easily from the grocery shops or supermarkets.)

2. Dissolve in a glass of chilled water.

3. Take it twice daily.

Note: For this vinegar and honey remedy, do not get commercial distilled vinegars as they do not contain the same health values of organic, raw apple cider vinegar. The powerful enzymes and minerals like potassium, phosphorus, sodium, magnesium, sulphur, iron copper, fluorine, silicon, pectin and natural malic and tartaric acids, which are important in fighting body toxins and inhibiting bacteria growth, are all destroyed during the distilling process.

Honey Cinnamon Fights Obesity and Many Other Health Problems

The combination of honey and cinnamon has been used in both oriental and Ayurvedic medicine for centuries. Cinnamon is one of the oldest spices known to mankind, while honey is an age-old food dating back thousands of years. The two ingredients with unique healing abilities have a long history as a home remedy. Cinnamon's essential oils and honey's enzyme that produces hydrogen peroxide qualify the two "anti-microbial" foods with the ability to help stop the growth of bacteria as well as fungi.
Both are used not just as a beverage flavouring and medicine, but also as an embalming agent and are used as alternatives to traditional food preservatives due to their effective antimicrobial properties.

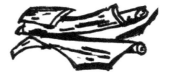

Many people have emailed me to share how this natural cure has worked wonders for high blood pressure, hypertension, high cholesterol level, bladder infection, asthma, acid reflux, constipation, and stomach ulcers, and described how the formula has brought about many health benefits, including improved digestion and weight loss. Though the mixture's taste can be distinctly nasty, many people have tolerated it and found the healing power of this mixture to be awe-inspiring. (Visit http://www.benefits-of-honey.com/honey-and-cinnamon.html to read testimonies on this alternative medicine.)

Weight Loss
The steps for preparing the honey and cinnamon concoction for losing weight are as follows:

1. Dissolve half a teaspoon of cinnamon powder (or ground cinnamon) in a cup of boiling water.

2. Stir and cover for half an hour.

3. Filter away any big particles and add a teaspoon of honey. (To keep the enzymes alive in honey, do not mix honey in hot water.)

4. Take it in the morning with an empty stomach about half an hour before breakfast. Repeat for the next three weeks or more to see results.

NOTES:
1. Many people are hesitant to try this concoction due to the intimidating prospect of eating cinnamon direct. I have tried it many times for general detoxification purposes and have found it to be especially helpful in moving bowel. And what do I say about the taste of this mixture? Pungent, spicy, and woody. The added honey definitely makes it a lot more palatable. My recommendation is, hold your breath and bring it down without thinking about the taste. In a minute, it's over.

2. Add honey only half an hour after mixing the cinnamon and boiling water, so that the healthy enzymes in the honey are kept alive.

34

Lowering Cholesterol

For preparing the home remedy for high blood pressure, hypertension, or high cholesterol level, follow these two steps:

1. Add in 2 tablespoon of pure honey and 1/8 tablespoon of cinnamon powder to a glass of warm water.

2. Mixed thoroughly and take the concoction first thing in the morning at least 30 minutes before your breakfast. Do not take anything (including water) before breakfast.

Relieving Joint Pains

Many honey enthusiasts have found honey and cinnamon to be especially effective for treating joint pains due to ailments such as rheumatoid arthritis.

In August 2009, a lady from Canada wrote to me, sharing that her brother-in-law had rheumatoid arthritis and had suffered many years of pain, swelling and discomfort. Apparently, he had tried many different pills prescribed by his doctor and nothing worked. So, he stopped all medication. Five years went past. His condition took for the worse, until one day, the lady's husband came to know about using honey to treat joint pain and swelling. He was given a print-out that instructed taking twice a day 2 tsp of honey and 1 tsp of cinnamon mixed with a cup of hot water. Her brother-in-law tried the recipe and within three days, he was amazed by the lack of pain he was feeling, and in no time, he was almost pain free.

In the same year, I received an email from another lady from Uganda who reported that for many years her husband was suffering from gout which would hit him anytime and anywhere. For every gout attack he had to go for inflammatory injection, until a friend advised them on the use of honey and cinnamon. He took it once a day in the morning and subsequently had not experienced a single attack again. Amazing story!

General Health
For bladder infections, stomach ulcer, asthma, acid reflux constipation, or as a general health remedy:

1. Add 2 teaspoons of pure honey and half a teaspoon of cinnamon powder to a cup of warm water or tea.

2. Take it daily.

Restoring Health & Losing Weight with The Hibernation Diet

Between 2007 and 2008, the Hibernation Diet created by a British pharmacist and a nutrition expert caught my attention by making a powerful connection between poor sleep and obesity. It advocates incorporating mild resistance exercise and a healthy, balanced, and wholesome diet void of highly refined, processed foods such as white bread, pizza, burgers, chocolates, beer and sugar, and suggests taking a generous spoonful or two of fructose-rich honey at night, either as a warm

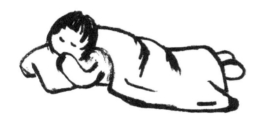

drink, a smoothie or straight from the jar.

Now, I expect what I just said to stir up an upheaval of emotions for many of you. How can something so sweet be any good when you are closely watching your weight? Doesn't it sound all too stupid to consume more calories before you sleep when you are trying all day to lose weight and reduce calories in your meals? Doesn't everyone know that our body metabolism rate at night is low, so we should avoid eating too late if we want a flat tummy? Surely, this defies common sense and must be one of those baseless old wives' tales about dieting or some quick fix that's central to all fad diets.

What you are going to read is going to transform your thinking about body metabolism, confront you to take quality sleep more seriously, and change the way you talk about this all-too-common golden liquid called, honey.

A revolutionary approach to fat metabolism, the Hibernation Diet believes that honey is the most ideal food that can provide a fuelling mechanism for the liver at night due to its 1:1 ratio of fructose to glucose. Mike McInnes, a pharmacist and the author of the Hibernation Diet, rediscovered the principles of human metabolism and the critical role of liver glycogen in recovery physiology that have been overlooked or ignored by the medical and sport science faculties.

As explained, our brain constitutes only 2% of our entire body mass, yet it's the most energy demanding organ, burning up to 20 times the fuel of any other cell in the body. And it can only store energy in a very restricted form. The liver is the only organ that can both store and release glucose for fuelling of the brain. Hence ensuring enough storage of liver glycogen amount during the 8 hours of night fasting is so critical. If we go to bed with a depleted liver, the brain triggers the release of stress hormones – adrenalin and cortisol in order to convert muscle protein into glucose required for the survival of the brain. And the overproduction of stress hormones not only works against our efforts to lose weight but in the long run (day after day, week after week, month after month...) can also lead to conditions such as obesity, heart disease, osteoporosis, diabetes, poor immune function, hypertension, depression and other distressing health problems.

Some simple questions that the hibernation diet expert asks to check if the liver has fuelled up well for the night:

- Do you wake regularly during the night?
- Do you have night sweats?
- Do you experience acid reflux during the night?
- Do you get up to go to the bathroom during the night?
- Do you feel nauseous in the early morning?
- Do you wake up exhausted?
- Do you have a dry throat in the morning?
- Do you get night cramps?
- Do you feel weak in the early morning?

If "yes" is the answer for any of these questions, it could mean that instead of burning fat and repairing muscles, your body has produced a stream of stress hormones while you sleep.

When talking about plans to lose weight, we have to understand that our body burn four types of fuel – body fats (adipose), fats within muscle tissue (triglycerides), glucose from liver glycogen, and glucose from muscle glycogen stores. The burning ratio during exercise or aerobics is 20% fat to 80% glucose. And during resting metabolism (sleep) this is reversed to 20% glucose and 80% fats!

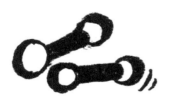

We have to know that body fat (adipose) is the fuel used to provide the energy of recovery physiology (sleep metabolism), and this fat is exclusively body and not muscle fat. Take for example, for a sedentary person who does not exercise, 2400 calories are required in 1 day (24 hrs) for survival. Thus metabolic rate is 100 calories/hr. Overnight consumption during 8 hrs of sleep is 800 calories. And if resting metabolism rate is 20% glucose and 80% fat, then during the night fast, 160 calories of glucose (in brain and red blood cells, mostly in brain) and 640 calories in fat (body fat) are utilised.

If this person visits a gym and expends 1000 calories, the ratio is 20% fat and 80% glucose, i.e. 200 calories of fat and 800 calories of glucose. In exercise, fat is sourced from both muscle fat (triglycerides) and body fat (adipose tissue) in equal amount. Thus the body fat consumed during exercise is only 100 calories, which is about only 11g or less than 0.5 ounce! In recovery state (during sleep), metabolism rate may be low, but it's healthy, and it burns body fats. Hence, if we focus only on measuring metabolism rates in our strife to lose weight, we miss the point.

The fact is, we cannot optimise body fat metabolism (20%:80%) overnight when we go to bed with a depleted liver. We activate stress hormones which inhibit glucose metabolism, which in turn undermines fat metabolism. The incredible news is, metabolism stress can be easily prevented by eating honey prior to bedtime as it provides adequate fuel for the liver during the night fast. Honey intelligently restocks the liver selectively without digestive burden and forms a stable supply of liver glycogen which our brain demands for the 8 hrs of night fast – when we sleep.

Central to the Hibernation Diet theory is the understanding of the role of sleep in restoring our body and health. Many people have the misconception that when we retire to bed, our body shuts down and goes to rest as well. The fact is, when we sleep, our body should go to work! Sleep is *"an energy-driven physiological process" and "a fat-burning physiology". The energy required during sleep for the brain and kidney must be sourced from the liver. Hence, to avoid metabolic stress and promote quality, restorative sleep, the liver has to be sufficiently restocked with honey before the night fast.

Thus far, I have received very inspiring testimonies about the positive effects of the Hibernation Diet. An Australian shared that he turned to the diet when he was diagnosed as prediabetic. After two years, he was able to sleep better, manage fatigue and depression better, and also experienced healing of his skin cancer. A Japanese also wrote to me, sharing how by following the hibernation diet has helped him lose a whopping 16kg over twenty months and reduced his triglyceride level in his blood from 585mg/dL to 157mg/dL without doing any exercises or changing his day-to-day eating habits. To read their full testimonies, I invite you to turn to: http://www.benefits-of-honey.com/hibernation-diet.html.

* Ron Fessenden & Mike McInnes (2008). The Honey Revolution. Restoring the Health of Future Generation. WorldClassEmprise, LLC.

Honey is Anti-Cancer

Honey is not an antidote for cancer or a "cure-all". But what many people have overlooked is - honey possesses carcinogen-preventing and anti-tumour properties.

Honey is curative and anti-cancer. According to the book Honey Revolution by Dr Ron Fessenden, scientists have found floral flavonoids in honey. These tiny traces of bioflavonoids, generally known as antioxidants, have powerful influences when entered into the body's cells. When ingested, they immediately increase the antioxidant levels within cells, "decrease capillary permeability and fragility. They scavenge oxidants and inhibit the destruction of collagen in the body". In fact in the recent years, major drug companies have recognised the effectiveness of these flora-flavones in removing free radicals from our body and improving our body immunity functioning, and are now investing millions of dollars just to produce these substances artificially.

Surely all of us know that prevention is far better than cures, but sadly, the world has succumbed to the instant gratification syndrome. Just see how people are losing weight so quickly by taking diet pills, getting liposuction, or even starving themselves. Working out things over time is considered as a waste of time. We want material wealth, relationships, and success immediately, totally abandoning the universal law of sowing and reaping. And with the exact attitude, we often put all our strength and focus into demanding instant cures of diseases and forget all about constant prevention.

Tell your family and friends that the foraging honeybees have passed on these precious natural floral-flavones from the floral nectars to honey and then to us! Look, you may not see the benefit of turning to healthful food overnight, but daily repetitive healthy choices will can potentially safe your life from deadly diseases like cancers.

My First Honey Water Fast

I had my first honey water fast experience in 2007; during the time I was beginning to uncover more and more exciting application of honey.

For six years after giving birth to two daughters, I was putting on a presumably insignificant kilo every year, until I scaled a weighty 66kg and realized that my wardrobe was changing far too fast and that standing at 1.66m with a protruding tummy was not at all flattering in any kind of outfit. Other than blaming it on my slow metabolism rate and a natural love for food, I discovered that there was surely more I could do – going on a diet. However, that was equally daunting. I was not ready to keep up with special diet plans and be involved in the preparation work for making special foods for each meal.

Then, one day while browsing in the library, I stumbled upon a Chinese book with the title "Slimming with Honey" (as I would translate it in the best possible way into English) written by a Taiwanese expert in Traditional Chinese Medicine. Being a new honey convert, I was naturally spurred to flip the pages to ascertain its usefulness. And when I read that the author lost 2kg and improved her skin complexion significantly in just three days by going a body detoxification program with honey and water as the only source of sustenance, I immediately checked the book out of the library.

I knew very well a 3-day fast was not a panacea that I could count on for weight problem, but I felt the hankering to put my body on a challenge for a few days of no food. And I figure that a detox could be a good jumpstart to get myself on the road of forming a better attitude towards eating and working on a wiser diet subsequently.

Yes, so I went on my very first 3-day detox, losing 3kg as a result (much of the weight was from water loss, I supposed). My tummy was reduced, my inner thighs didn't seem to rub against each other so much anymore when I walk, and I felt lighter, and could even fit into some of my old clothing.

The beauty of this 3-day program is its simplicity – no complicated diet plans to follow from Monday to Sunday, nor any fat-burning pills to pop, or any creams or ointment to rub on the tummy regularly. What it requires only are the availability of pure honey, a resolution to abstain from food for three days and a correct attitude when breaking fast. Knowing how nutritious honey is helps in bracing me up for the program. I was convinced that this natural sweetener containing a myriad of small doses of nutrients and vitamins and a horde of antioxidants is a wise choice of food during this time. But what probably also inspired me a great deal is the well-known proposition that our organs occasionally deserve a good break after working so hard non-stop since the day we were born and allowed ourselves to indulge in the immensity of so-called good foods. Moreover fasting isn't a rocket science; for thousands of years, almost all cultures have counted on it to help clear the body of toxins, give our digestive organs the opportunity to rejuvenate and restore optimum function.

This Honey Water Detoxification simply involves the following: For 3 days, take only honey with water or tea. For each 150cc of water, mix with 1 to 2 tablespoons of pure honey. Drink this for breakfast, lunch and dinner, and whenever you feel tired or thirsty. Keep yourself hydrated the whole day but limit total consumption of honey to 150cc each day.

Day One:

The temptation for food and to give it up and start all over again was very real for me. I constantly felt hunger pangs and my mind just kept slipping into images of my favourite foods. However, reminding myself of what the book shared – "one should get used to it on the 2nd day" gave me great consolation and courage to stay on. Focusing on my work in the office nonetheless was a big challenge when every nerve and cell in me was screaming for food.

Day Two:

As per what was described in the book, I experienced more energy instead of weakness and an improved bowel movement. However, what was disappointing to me was – there was no euphoria high as I continued to fast and my yearning for food did not seem to get any lesser. I somehow didn't get used to hunger like how the book has described and all I wanted to do when I got back home from work was to sleep and shut out any ill-feelings.

Day Three:

I was a bit surprised by my energy level in the morning and happy that I could still keep up with my usual 30-minute workout at 6.30am. And thankfully, my gastric did not give me any problems like in the past whenever I skipped meals. However, by noon, I was feeling famished again and by 5pm I was actually getting upset and moody about the depravity of food. And one strange phenomenon that was really not funny - I became extremely sensitive to odours and even the smell of people's breath! To brighten up things a bit on my last day of fasting, I expanded the range of tea varieties that I use to chamomile, rose, and fruit, and also increase the floral varieties of honey to Clover, Leatherwood, and Manuka. By evening, when I stepped onto my bathroom scale, I had already lost an unbelievable 3kg and a big bulk of my tummy.

Day Four:

To break fast, I followed the author's advice of going on a soft diet and abstaining from meat, dairy products, and oily and spicy stuff for the first two days. My breakfast consisted of a small bowl of oat cereal mixed with honey, but to my surprise, I didn't feel excited at all when I tasted food again. In the afternoon, I was hungry and eager to go for some nice soft food but at the same time also felt somewhat revolting. Eating seemed to be a brand new experience. Flavours and textures of foods had become so different for me that I actually could not appreciate their tastes like before. My appetite was so bad that it was almost like having dreadful symptoms of morning sickness. In the end, I ended eating only a slice of fresh papaya, half a bowl of plain congee, a cup of water melon juice, and honey water for the whole day. Only then did I realise that breaking fast was even be harder than fasting itself.

Day Five:

The start of the day was not as depressing as the day before. I began to respond to food more positively and continued to take bland, soft food. By evening, to my relief, my appetite was back to normal and that was when I did something stupid – I gluttonously gulped down a bottle of cold lemon juice to quench my thirst. And result? I ended the day with a big mess, whining like a baby, throwing up big time and feeling weak. What a memorable anti-climax to my fasting experience!

Day Six:

I slowly normalized my diet, but still avoiding food that is too sweet, sour and spicy, or salty, so that my stomach could slowly get used to having different types of foods again.

12 Things I Learnt From This Honey Water Fast:

1. Take only pure, unadulterated honey. Raw honey which is the most nutritious form of honey of course is the best. Use it if it's available.

2. Make use of different honey varieties and assorted tea types to make the 3-day fast less dreadful.

3. Stay away from icy cold water, strongly caffeinated teas such as red tea, and oolong tea, alcohol and don't smoke.

4. Do not add to your tea and honey any lemon, which can be too hard and stimulating for the stomach. Take just water, and soothing honey and tea.

5. Following an amazing theory in the hibernation diet which I had previously read, I take a glass of warm honey drink before going to bed so as to fuel the liver, speed up fat-burning metabolism, and keep blood sugar levels balanced.

6. You could modify this three-day program to two days or one day, or even one meal to suit your needs. For instance, on occasions when you feel you have overeaten, you might wish to detoxify the body for a day by replacing all foods with just honey drinks.

7. I wouldn't recommend this diet for young children, pregnant mothers, and people with a medical condition. If you are ill or recuperating from a sickness, postpone your fasting.

8. This detox program is so easy that I feel it could also be very suitable for men who are trying to lose weight but would not bother a bit to figure out how to prepare all the special meals, or have no time or energy to do so.

9. Whenever you are about to give up while fasting because you feel you could not withstand the hunger, tell yourself that it is really possible and you can make it. If others can do it, so can you. Always go back to your initial intention – what makes you want to do this. Picture yourself in the desired state of health, distract yourself with lots of things to do, and persevere.

10. Remember that fasting is not complete without proper breaking of the fast – which is just as important and can be even harder. Be mentally prepared to put up a fight when confronting food again because a slumbering digestive system is highly sensitive and needs time to get back to speed. Take fresh fruit and vegetables slowly and drink fresh fruit juices. Avoid cold and citrus stuff. Eat smaller meals, chew your food well, and eat according to hunger. My fast-breaking experience confirmed what the book has forewarned – do not lose control and overeat, do not jar the digestive system by gorging on meat and junk food.

11. I took 2 days to break the 3-day honey water detox. The rule of thumb is: the longer the fast, the more time is needed for breaking the fast. Typically, a period of no less than one half the length of the fast is required for breaking the fast. Going through a disciplined re-feeding process helps me reinforce good dietary habits and now I seem to be more conscious of what I eat.

12. Finally, it is erroneous thinking that you can eat all you want after you have deprived yourself for a while. We need to get this right: Fasting is not a cure for obesity or any sickness; it is a process that facilitates the body's own healing mechanism. Rightly conducted, it is a sure, quick, safe way to unload a toxic overload. Abstinence from food, followed by rational eating, has proven to be very effective in helping thousands to give up bad eating habits, re-establish health and strength.

Nature's First Aid Burn Treatment

If you ever get burnt, run to honey for cure.

What honey can do as a burn treatment has always been head knowledge until 13 April 2009 when unfortunately I had to experience it myself. Reports about honey as a home remedy for burns from honey enthusiasts have always left me so bowled over, and then now after beholding what honey could do for scalded skin, I had to cry out "What it's been said is really true!" I was so wowed by the fact that nature had bestowed upon us such an extraordinary medicine.

The incident happened during dinner time while I was lading boiling soup into bowls for my children. Carelessly, I swirled the bowl slightly, causing a few drops of the soup to fall unto my right palm, and because I was so startled by the unexpected hot sensation, I jolted and caused a further spillage of the soup on my entire palm.

My very first instinct was to run for the basin and put my scalded hand under the running tap. The pain set in instantly and slowly became excruciating. In a frenzy of anxiety, I raced to grab a tube of burn cream from the fridge and apply it on my palm. In spite of that, the pain became even more intense, and my palm turned red.

That was when I was reminded of the wonders of honey.

Frantically, I washed off the cream and scooped a teaspoon of honey from the jar to rub on my palm. With this, a warm sensation came on the skin. In no more than five minutes, the throbbing pain left! After leaving the honey on for about half an hour and then washing it off, my skin initially felt some numbness, but everything returned to normal in just minutes. There was not a sign of burn on my palm; neither blisters nor redness. I was perfectly well!

Since then, I would recall that fateful incident whenever I sustained a burn. And every time, honey worked like magic. It has to be the best burn ointment nature has given to us!

If you want to read about other amazing real stories of using honey as a superb ointment for hot oven burns, hot soup burns, hot hair curling iron, and hot oil, go to: http://www.benefits-of-honey.com/the-benefits-of-honey.html. Here's one which I would particularly like to mention because it's so powerful – A girl in high school burned her face with the curling iron while trying to answer the phone. She became so desperate when the wound turned brown and everyone started asking her what happened. Her cousin instructed her to apply raw honey, and in a few days, her skin was healed, leaving behind not a single scar.

Honey Skin Care

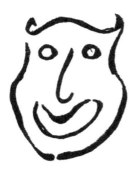

Honey is a great natural anti-aging skin care product.

Throughout the centuries, legendary beauties like Cleopatra and Poppea, wife of Roman Emperor Nero have used raw honey as part of their skin and hair care treatments to keep them looking youthful.

This natural healing agent contains an enzyme called glucose oxidase, that when combined with water, produces hydrogen peroxide, a mild antiseptic. In addition to the glucose oxidase enzyme, honey also contains antioxidants and flavonoids that may function as antibacterial agents. It is a humectant, having the ability attract and retain moisture, and to rebuild the moisture level in the skin without making it oily. As a natural moisturiser, it helps replenish necessary skin moisture, especially during the winter months (for those who experience different seasons). This is why honey is a popular anti aging skin care ingredient in many commercial moisturizing products including cleansers, creams, shampoos, shower gels, and conditioners. And because it's so gentle, it is suitable for sensitive skin and popularly used in baby care products.

I've listed down some of the most popular facial mask recipes for different skin types. In fact because so many honey buffs have become so excited by the results and are even making some for their neighbours and friends, I believe you will appreciate them too.

For Dry Skin: Avocado & Honey Face Mask:

You will need:
2 tablespoons of avocado flesh
2 tablespoons honey
1 egg yolk

To form this anti aging skin care face mask, put all the ingredients in a blender, or mash by hand in a bowl. Use your fingers to spread the mask over your face and neck and leave it on for 30-50 minutes before removing.

For Dry Skin: Honey and Egg Mask:

You will need
1 tablespoon honey
1 egg yolk
1/2 teaspoon almond oil
1 tablespoon yogurt

Put all ingredients into a large bowl and stir until it becomes sticky and thick. Apply the mask to your face for 5 minutes and wash face thoroughly with a mild facial soap. Honey stimulates and smoothes, egg and almond oil penetrate and moisturize, and yogurt refines and tightens pores.

For Tired Skin: Almond Yoghurt Honey Mask

You will need:
6oz plain yoghurt
¼oz finely-crushed almonds
2tsp honey
2tsp wheat germ oil

Mix all the ingredients into a smooth paste. Apply and massage the mixture into skin. Keep the mask on for 20 minutes.

For Normal Skin: Apple Honey Mask

You will need
1 Apple, cored & quartered
2 Tablespoons Honey
Drop the apple pieces into a food processor and chop. Add honey and refrigerate for 10 minutes. Pat the mixture onto your face with a light tapping motion, tapping until the honey feels tacky. Leave it on for 30 minutes and then rinse.

For Oily Skin: Honey-Papaya Mask

You will need:
1/3-cup cocoa
3 teaspoons of heavy cream
1/3-cup ripe papaya
1/4-cup honey and 3 teaspoons of oatmeal powder

Mix and apply on your face. After 10 minutes, wash your face with warm water. This anti aging skin care face mask helps heal skin blemishes, nourishes, draws out impurities, balances your skin pH, and will leave your skin radiant and soft. Good for acne-prone skin.

For Oily Skin: Carrot Face Mask

Your will need
2-3 carrots
4 1/2 table spoons of honey

Cook the carrots and then mash them up. Mix the carrots with honey and refrigerate for 10 minutes. Apply gently to the skin and wait for ten minutes. Rinse off with cool water. Carrots are known to be rich in Vitamin A and C. They are also rich in potassium. Honey contains enzymes, minerals, vitamins and amino acids.

For Sensitive Skin: Banana and Honey Mask

You will need
1/2 mashed banana
1/4 cup oatmeal, cooked with milk
1 egg
1/2 tablespoon honey

Mix ingredients together. Massage onto face in a slow, circular motion and leave for 15 minutes. Rinse with tepid water. Oatmeal is high in nourishing vitamins and minerals; it gently cleanses and heals skin. Bananas contain Vitamin A; eggs contain lecithin, a natural skin emollient; and honey helps to maintain the skin's natural acid mantle.

For All Skin Types: Honey and Lavender Facial Mask

You will need:
1 tablespoon raw honey
3 drops lavender essential oil

Mix the ingredients, dampen your face with warm water, and smooth on the honey and lavender mixture. Leave the mask on for 15 minutes. Then rinse off with warm water.

If all the above recipes are far too complicated for you to prepare, consider applying just raw honey plus a little salt as a facial mask. According to many, this helps keep out blackheads and smoothen the skin.

More Health Benefits of Honey

Adding to my conviction that honey must be differentiated from other sugars are the stories that come streaming continually through my website. Below are extracted snippets of testimonies about how the precious liquid had contributed to the healing of the body.

Veinus Ulcers:
"I currently use raw honey as an alternative to doctor prescribed medicines containing silver for the treatment of veinus ulcers in my lower legs. Alternating honey and the prescribed drugs, I have found that healing is elevated several times faster than just prescribed medicines..."

Poor Eyesight:
"Every morning, I mix honey with carrot juice to improve my eyesight..."

Fatigue:
"What's most important for me is the anabolic properties of honey. Raw honey seems to help me maintain muscle, have less fatigue, and tolerate cold better. These things are all related to a more anabolic condition in the body..."

Chapped Lip:
"...apply some honey on your lips at night before you sleep to have this fabulous pink lips! My friends recommended this to me because my lips were always chapped and pale..."

Wart:
"I told a friend about the honey-wart cure. She was on the way to taking her son to the doctor to have numerous seed warts burned off her son's knee. She applied the honey, wrapped the knee with gauze. About a half hour later, her son took a shower in preparation of his doctor's visit. The warts were all washed off in the shower. The doctor's visit was cancelled..."

Hair Loss:
"My mother-in-law suffered from Alopecia (hair loss disease) and I told her about the honey/cinnamon/hot olive oil recipe for hair loss and her hair has grown back. Her doctor is shocked. He had her on prescription medication and topical shampoos that had little or no effect."

Surely, honey protects and prevents diseases. When consumed regularly, honey is able to reverse many negative health trends. The amazing health benefits of honey go beyond our comprehension. Some of the benefits can be experienced in a matter of days or weeks; others may take months or years to be appreciated. If only more would believe in taking honey consistently and continually, day after day...

The Honey Allergy Debate

Does honey allergy exist? Can honey cause allergic reactions since an amount of pollen from the plants that the honey nectar is gathered from could possibly be found in honey?

While extolling the benefits of honey, I have received emails from people who had reported reactions from ingesting even a drop of honey, and these include compulsory vomiting, stomach cramps, bloatedness, nausea, asthma, breathlessness, burning lips, itching ears itch, swelling throat, and chest pains. A few furious people also sent unfriendly emails to claim that eating a teaspoon would kill them.

I wouldn't dismiss honey allergies, but as it seems, serious reactions in pollen-allergic patients challenged with honey are rare.

I am no expert in allergies. As per my usual advice to my readers, a medical doctor's diagnosis should always be sought for any perceived honey allergy. Nonetheless, we all know that proteins are connected to most food allergies. Honey itself is mainly simple sugars, which are carbohydrates and do not cause allergic responses.

Commercially produced honey is filtered and pasteurized (sometimes even diluted with syrup), hence the amount of bee pollen in the honey is probably low. And if you are concerned about honey allergy issues, please do consult your doctor. Unprocessed raw honey may contain residual proteins which are pollens from the plants the bees visited, and pollens are a well-known, established allergen (not honey itself). For people who are sensitive to pollens, they ought to be very cautious about taking not just honey, but any other bee products such as propolis, royal jelly, and raw honey (example eating honey straight from honeycomb), nobody could really guarantee the absence of pollens in those bee products. In fact, for these people, they have to be exceptionally careful of any food they eat as honey could be an ingredient in all sorts of foods, including flavoured drinks, bread, pastries, cakes, chocolate, candy bars, and cereals.

A honey retailer in Singapore shared with me that none of her customers had complained of allergic reactions, but some had experienced temporary setbacks like body ache, fever, flu, diarrhoea or breaking a lot of wind (farting). All of them recovered after a few days. She believed that such reactions were normal as the honey was working and the body was reacting to its various healing effects. It was advised that one could continue but in smaller doses when such "allergic-like" reaction developed in the initial stages, and if the honey quality was not a suspect, the "allergies" would disappear after a few days.

Hence, I do not dismiss "honey allergy", but I tend to believe that it would not be right to list honey as an allergen alongside with pollen, bee venom (from bee stings), dust, or food-based allergens like peanuts, eggs, milk, nuts, and shellfish. The safety concern about honey could also have arisen because of the presence of spores that are able to cause a rare deadly disease discovered in 1976, called infant botulism. While honey allergies cannot be 100% established and we all know that consumption of honey is generally safe for adults, many people actually believe that eating local honey could counteract and treat allergies to these pollens by helping the body to become tolerant of them. That is, honey acts as an immune booster against the allergies. The good effects of this local honey are best when the honey is taken a little bit (a couple of teaspoons-full) a day for several months prior to the pollen season. It is said that the closer the honey is raised to where you live, the better it is.

Thomas Leo Ogren of "Allergy-Free Gardening" says, "It may seem odd that straight exposure to pollen often triggers allergies but that exposure to pollen in the honey usually has the opposite effect. But this is typically what we see. In honey the allergens are delivered in small, manageable doses and the effect over time is very much like that from undergoing a whole series of allergy immunology injections. The major difference though is that the honey is a lot easier to take and it is certainly a lot less expensive. I am always surprised that this powerful health benefit of local honey is not more widely understood, as it is simple, easy, and often surprisingly effective."

 If you decide to give the local honey a try to treat allergies, consult your physician before use.

I'm Diabetic, Can I Eat Honey?

The diabetic diet is strictly controlled in terms of sugar and mineral compounds intake. Hence it's not surprising that diabetic patients frequently ask if they are allowed to eat honey.

Clinical studies have shown that pure honey is a healthier choice in diabetic diet than table sugar and other non-nutritive sweeteners such as Splenda, saccharin, aspartame. Honey requires lower levels of insulin compared to regular white sugar and does not raise blood sugar levels as rapidly as table sugar, that is, it has a lower Glycemic Index than sugar. Although honey contains a significant amount of sugar, it consists largely of two simple individual units of sugar - glucose and fructose, which are absorbed at different rates into the body.

With appropriate control, many diabetics and pre-diabetes (people with blood glucose levels higher than normal person but not high enough to be considered diabetic) are still able to safely enjoy natural honey. However, they should first consult their doctor or dietician before incorporating honey into their meal planning and find out how much honey can be consumed on a daily basis. Each diabetic is different and has to learn how his or her body reacts to different foods containing carbohydrates. Bear in mind that the total amount of starches or carbohydrates in a food is the key consideration, not the amount of sugar. Honey is a carb food as well, just like rice and potatoes. Thus just keep in mind that 1 tablespoon of honey has approximately 17 grams of carbohydrate, and taking that into account when counting your total daily intake of carbohydrates, diabetics can work it out just like any other sweetener or carbohydrates. One way of determining if honey is right for you is to test your blood sugar levels before you eat it and again two hours later. Also, when purchasing commercial honey for diabetic patients, be sure that it is pure and not adulterated by glucose, starch, cane sugar, and even malt, which are all better to be avoided in a diabetic diet.

Why Babies Should Not Be Given Honey?
Any Warning for Pregnant Mothers?

For whatever reason or purpose, do not give honey to infants under the age of 18 months (to be on the safer side, though some doctors would say 12 months).

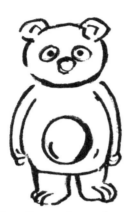

Some honey contains low count of naturally occurring bacterial botulinum spores, which bees collect together with the nectar. These spores cannot be removed during honey processing and cannot be detected by consumers. A baby's immature digestive system is not yet acidic enough to inhibit the toxin from being produced, whereas the digestive system of an older baby and adults is. Hence, there is a potential for these organism to thrive and grow in the intestines of young infant's intestines and produce toxin, possibly causing a serious form of food poisoning known as infant botulism. The typical symptoms of this illness are constipation followed by general weakness and poor feeding ability.

How about a pregnant mom or a nursing mom? The digestive tract of adults is able to fend off the botulism spores, render them harmless, and prevent them from growing. Since the spores would be killed in the gastrointestinal tract, no toxin will be produced to endanger the foetus of the pregnant mother. Similarly, for nursing mothers, these spores would not make it into your bloodstream and therefore cannot be present in their milk. In fact, milk with honey is good and safe for pregnant women who are desperate to get a good night's sleep or are troubled by heartburn sensations. And ginger tea with honey is a great remedy for nausea and vomiting.

Are all Honey Varieties Equal?

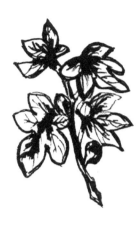

Some people judge honey quality by their floral origin, but each floral variety has its own distinct and original taste, texture, and color. Flavors vary from very mild and bland to strong and pungent and colors range from dark brown to colorless. Color is used in the honey industry as a convenient measure of honey flavour and aroma. As a general rule of thumb, light-colored honey is milder in taste and dark-colored honey, more robust.

The unique aroma and colour of each of the honey varieties are determined by the floral source, such as clover, basswood, orange blossom or buckwheat, from which the bee collects the nectar. Aristotle the Greek philosopher reported in the 3rd century B.C that honey bees which have gathered from a certain flower choose to return to another flower of the same sort and they communicate to other foreigners in the hive by means of scent and physical movement, the location of the specific nectar source. He observed that on each expedition the bee does not fly from a flower of one kind to a flower of another kind until it has got back to the hive. On reaching the hive, the bees throw off their load and each bee on her return is followed by three or four companions. Bees can select the best yielding nectar source available at a given time, which leads them to concentrate on a single source. Hives that have been moved into blooming fields for purposes of pollination offer bees a great single source to collect from. In order to be labelled as a certain variety, a honey must be 80% from the named source.

Honey varies not only in colour and flavour, but also in its medicinal properties, with some varieties such as New Zealand's Manuka honey and Malaysia's Tualang honey being more potent than others. After trying out so many different brands of honey, I find that the same floral variety of honey of different brands may not taste exactly the same. Climatic conditions of the area can influence the colour, quality, and thus flavour and taste of honey varieties.

UMF Manuka Honey

Unique Manuka Factor or commonly known as UMF is the only worldwide standard in identifying and measuring the antibacterial strength or quality of some strains of Manuka. It is a guarantee that the honey being sold has the special UMF antibacterial property and a UMF rating of 10 is the minimum recognised. While ordinary Manuka has only the hydrogen peroxide antibacterial property which is common to most types of honey, UMF Manuka has both the natural hydrogen peroxide antibacterial property and its own natural UMF antibacterial property, giving it increased antibacterial potency. The UMF property is very stable, unlike the hydrogen peroxide antibacterial property common in most honey which is easily destroyed by heat, light as well as certain enzymes in body serum.

UMF Manuka, also known as "Medihoney" in some pharmacies, is the preferred honey for wound dressing and other special therapeutic uses. Studies have shown that Manuka with high levels of UMF could be very effective in helping relieve stomach ulcer symptoms and gastritis, and sore throats, and when applied topically, in assisting the natural cure of skin ulcers, wounds, burns, boils, cracked skin. That is also why many skincare products also contain UMF Manuka as a special ingredient and promise positive benefits from their regular application on the skin.

A few specific uses of this honey for hair and skin problems are stated below:

Hair fall:
"Make a paste by mixing olive oil, 1 tablespoon of Manuka honey and 1 teaspoon of cinnamon powder. Massage on the scalp and leave it for 15-20 minutes. Wash off and repeat it for 3-4 times a week."

Seborrheic dermatitis:
"Dab the Manuka honey directly on the affected skin. Repeat daily for 1-2 weeks."

Acne skin:
"Mix three tablespoons of Manuka honey together with one teaspoon of cinnamon to get rid of pimples before they can cause acne scars. Apply the honey cinnamon paste as a facial mask and leave it on for 1 hour before washing it off with warm water. Repeat this acne treatment for two week."

UMF is not found in the nectar of all Manuka flowers, which are known as Leptospermum Scoparium and belong to the Tea Tree bushes found only in New Zealand's coastal areas. Some Manuka bushes do not produce honey with the UMF property every year, and the concentrations of UMF can vary from batch to batch and year to year. The reason why only some Manuka honeys have the unique UMF antibacterial property is not yet known. Researchers believe that it could be from a subspecies of Manuka or due to some environmental factor such as soil type.

There are varying UMF strengths - UMF 10, UMF 15, UMF 20, UMF 25, and the higher the UMF, the more expensive is the honey. All genuine UMF Manuka honeys from New Zealand are packed into jars and labelled with a registered trademark UMF® by licensed companies, and have a rating of UMF 10 or more. These licensed users of the UMF® label in New Zealand have to meet standards of regular monitoring and auditing of their honey quality. So if you come across an UMF honey which is packed in New Zealand and is labelled UMF 8, you should know something is amiss. Another reason why Manuka honey, which is available in most Kiwi homes, is favoured by so many honey buffs is that it has a higher than normal conductivity, which is an indirect measurement of mineral content of a honey -- about four times that of normal flower honeys.

The taste of Manuka is probably an acquired one; the more I eat it, the more I can appreciate its remarkable depth and unique forest aroma that stands out amongst the honey varieties. I love everything about it except its price. Laboratory testing and licensing fees for the use of the UMF trademark probably are key drivers of UMF Manuka's exorbitant price. A UMF labelled bottle of Manuka honey in Singapore is about 10 times or more the price of regular honey! Alternatively, there is relatively cheaper Manuka honey that makes no UMF claim, but the flipside is you wouldn't have a clue about its antibacterial strength.

Forms and Types of Honey

Raw honey versus commercial honey:

Raw honey is the concentrated nectar of flowers that comes straight from the extractor; it is the only unheated, pure, unpasteurized, unprocessed honey. Most honey found in the supermarket is not raw honey but "commercial" honey, which has been heated and filtered so that it looks cleaner and smoother, more appealing on the shelf, and easier to handle and package. When honey is heated, its delicate aromas, yeast and enzymes which are responsible for activating vitamins and minerals in the body system are partially destroyed. Hence, such honey is not as nutritious as raw honey.

Characterised by fine textured crystals, raw honey looks milkier and contains particles and flecks made of bee pollen, honeycomb bits, propolis, and broken bee wing fragments. Raw and unfiltered honey is relatively low in moisture content (14% to 18%) and has a high antioxidant level. It will usually granulate and crystallize to a margarine-like consistency after a month or two. Many people prefer to spread it on bread and waffles, dissolve it in hot coffee or tea, or use it for cooking and baking.

Among manufacturers there exists no uniform code of using the term "raw honey". There are no strict legal requirements for claiming and labelling honey as "raw". You may find raw honey that are unprocessed but slightly warmed to retard granulation for a short period of time and allow light straining and packing into containers for sale. In this case, the honey will not be considered 100% "raw" because it has been heated slightly and therefore rightfully should not be labelled as such by the supplier. Using as little heat as possible is a sign of careful handling.

Honey is differentiated by its physical form - comb, liquid, or cream, with each offering a different experience in terms of tasting.

1. Comb honey:

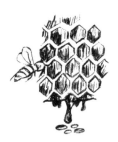

It is difficult to find comb honey from the stores nowadays, but sometimes you can find jars of liquid honey to which a piece of cut comb has been added. Before the invention of honey extracting device, honey is mostly produced in the form of comb honey. Today, very little honey is produced as comb honey.

Comb honey is raw pure honey sections taken straight from the hive – honey bees' wax comb with no further handling at all. It is the most unprocessed form in which honey comes -- the bees fill the hexagon shaped wax cells of the comb with honey and cap it with beeswax. You can eat comb honey just like a chewy candy.

Because the honey in the comb is untouched and is deemed to be pure, honey presented and marketed in this form comes with a relatively higher price tag.

2. Liquid honey:

Found everywhere easily, liquid honey has been filtered to remove fine particles, pollen grains, and air bubbles, and heated to melt visible crystals after being extracted from the honey comb by centrifugal force or gravity. Because liquid honey mixes easily into a variety of foods, its uses are diverse. It is used as a syrup for pancakes and waffles and in a wide variety of recipes, and is especially convenient for cooking and baking.

3. Cream honey:

If you are one of those who complain that honey is messy to use, cream honey, which is also known as whipped honey, spun honey, granulated honey, or honey fondant, would be an excellent alternative to liquid honey. As the crystallisation process has been controlled very precisely, cream honey does not drip like liquid honey, has a smooth consistency and can be spread like butter. (Note: This form of honey is sometimes erroneously perceived by some people as "pure, unadulterated honey" due to its viscosity, which we know is not a correct measurement of purity for honey.)

It has one part finely granulated honey blended with nine parts liquid honey. Crystallisation lightens the color of honey, but does not affect the taste and nutritional goodness at all. For instance, creamed premium lavender honey from the south of France is white in the jar. For those who live in warm climate countries like me, you probably might have noticed that the creamed honey that you buy from the air-conditioned super-mart becomes darker in colour and runnier when placed in room temperature.

Note: Honey does not remain stable if the moisture content is too high. No reputable honey supplier would add water to honey, as this would cause the honey to ferment and emit an alcoholic smell.

What is "Pure Honey"?

Many people ask how we could differentiate 100% pure honey and adulterated honey. I would like to share my experience and thoughts on this from a honey consumer's perspective.

The term "adulterated honey" implies that the honey has been added glucose, dextrose, molasses, corn syrup, sugar syrup, invert sugar, flour, starch, or any other similar product, other than the floral nectar gathered, processed, and stored in the comb by honey bees. Legal standards and requirements for foods, including honey quality, and tests for honey adulteration vary widely amongst countries and some may not meet the wish of every consumer around the world.

Most ideally, for the peace of mind, personally purchase fresh honey directly from your local beekeepers. However, if you do not have the privilege of being located near any bee farm like me, my take is always -- go for the trusted or more known brands. Personally, when selecting honey in the shop, I think it's impossible to tell the bad from the good by just looking at the honey content through the bottle or studying its food and nutrition labels. We all know that a "pure honey" label does not guarantee at all that it is not diluted with water and further sweetened with corn syrup; it just promises that there is real pure honey inside, with no suggestion of its amount. The law does not require a "pure honey" label to say how much pure honey is in the bottle. Also, prices are not always a good indication of quality honey. In food fraud cases, manufacturers can mix different honey floral blends and sell it as more expensive varieties such as Manuka honey. And so-called "local honey" may not be locally produced and processed local honey but cheap, low quality honey imported from other countries and then bottled and distributed locally.

It is a common misconception that granulation or crystallization of honey is a sign of adulteration with sugar water. The truth is honey is a supersaturated sugar solution and can granulate whether or not it has been adulterated. Crystallization is normal, especially in temperate climates. Furthermore, some honey from certain floral sources is especially prone to crystallization.

It is hard to be really absolutely sure about honey authenticity, unless from home you can perform scientific laboratory test like spectroscopy, a method that uses the principle of interaction of light with mater to differentiate substances or conduct carbon isotope ratios analysis to determine if sugars were added to the honey. Buying honey in the comb is one way to assure ourselves of a quality product as comb honey is sealed in the hive by the bees and cannot be adulterated.

How Much Honey is Excessive?

How much honey can we eat every day? What would be considered as excessive dosage?

I apply a general rule of thumb to my own personal consumption - not more than 10 teaspoons of honey (which is about 50ml) per day. Please note that this is not formulated by any medical point of view or scientific data.

I would expect the amount of honey considered to be optimum to depend a whole lot on a person's weight (adults versus children), diet and lifestyle. For instance, one could be taking foods with very low sugar content every day, leading a very active lifestyle, and following a disciplined exercise regimen, while on the other extreme end; another with a sweet tooth could be taking plenty of high-sugar stuff and living a sedentary lifestyle. Hence, apparently, the daily amount of honey to be prescribed for different people would not be the same.

As per the widely-known principle, excessiveness of any food, including honey is not wise. But note, not all sweeteners are equal. One excellent way to healthier eating is to use honey in our everyday food, for example, replace empty-calorie table sugar with nutritious honey in your routine beverages, spread honey instead of jam on bread, etc, For instance, if all this while you have been taking tea, coffee, or juices with table sugar in all your regular meals, you could straight away replace the sugar with honey. Some people have another concern about honey, that is, if eating honey, a very sweet liquid, would cause them to gain weight. Actually, the principle of weight gain is very simple: When you eat more than what your body needs, regardless of whether it is sugar, fat, or honey, the excess calories are stored as fat which in turns leads to weight gain.

If you are doing a full fasting, taking in only liquids and no other foods (which is not a normal diet), I learned from a honey fast book that an average-size adult could take up to about 150ml to 200ml honey mixed with water or tea everyday for a few days. This recommendation is for a full-fasting that lasts only a few days with just honey water for detoxification purposes. The only source of carbohydrate/energy during the fast is the honey consumed. Hence, the daily honey dosage for such a fast could look something like – two glasses of water/tea each time with a tablespoon of honey (about 15ml) each, for breakfast, lunch, at 3pm, dinner, and before bedtime. All these would add up to about 150ml of honey in total for a day.

How to Best Store Honey?

It was reported that archaeologists found 2000 year old jars of honey in Egyptian tombs and they still tasted delicious!

Honey is a miracle food; it never goes bad! Many people find it rather surprising that bacteria cannot grow in honey because all things being equal, bacteria love sugar. The unique chemical composition of low water content and relatively high acidic level in honey creates a low pH (3.2-4.5) environment that makes it very unfavourable for bacteria or other micro-organism to grow.

Since honey doesn't spoil even without any preservatives and additives, the "Best Before Dates" on honey buckets indicating its shelf life do not seem to be of any importance then. However, liquid honey is susceptible to physical and chemical changes during storage; it tends to darken and lose some of its aroma and flavour. Over time, liquid honey also tends to naturally crystallise and become lumpy. Crystallisation is easily reversible and does not affect the taste and quality of the honey at all, although it changes its appearance. Hence, for commercial reasons, a certain shelf life is often stated on the honey bottles in the shop.

All nectar contains some kind of yeast which can reproduce in higher-moisture content honey and cause fermentation. While fermentation does not necessarily pose any health risk, some manufacturers do pasteurization whereby the honey is heated very quickly to kill any yeast cell without damaging the product too much and then rapidly cooled. Pasteurized honey also has a slower granulation process and will last longer in its liquid state.

It is often read in honey storage tips that honey has to be kept at room temperature and should neither be stored in too cold nor too hot place. The question is "What is room temperature?" Doesn't it vary from country to country? For instance, where I live, room temperature sometimes could be as high as 35°C but I do not refrigerate any of my honey as cold temperatures would speed up the process of granulation.

Honey should ideally be stored in a cool, dry place. Make sure that the cap is on tight as honey tends to absorb moisture from the environment, which can lower its quality. Also store honey away from direct sunlight as it could affect its properties. This is the reason why some honey comes in dark containers, which however, do not allow consumers to judge the colour, viscosity, clarity, and crystallisation of the honey.

The rate of crystallisation varies for the different types of honey. Tupelo honey and Acacia honey, for instance, tend to stay liquid and is able to resist crystallisation better than other types of honey, whereas Lavender honey rushes to crystallise. Honey that has been processed and heated will remain liquid for a few months. Nevertheless, it's easy to restore granulated honey to its natural state, for instance you could put grainy honey on hot toast, and the granules will melt as you eat. You can also place a granulated jar over hot water (about 50-60°C), as soon as the granules are dissolved, remove the honey from the heat and let it cool as quickly as possible. Remember, never boil honey!

Honey in Singapore

"I live in a tiny country where there are no bee farms, no beekeepers, no beekeeping activities; I hardly see any bees buzzing around nor learn about any local allergies due to pollen..."

"Where on earth could this be?"

Singapore, a geographically small, modern, prosperous island-city-state in South-eastern Asia located at the tip of the Malaysian Peninsular, is where I reside. Ironically, it is also known as the Garden City famous for its wealth of flora and fauna, and it is one of the world's largest importers and exporters of honey.

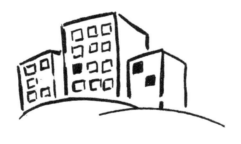

There is not a single honey bee farm or beekeeping activity in Singapore, and needless to say, no local beekeeping associations where beekeepers share information with the public. I do not know of any efforts to enlist honey manufacturers to promote and talk about the health and taste benefits of honey in Singapore. And never have I seen an in-store cooking demonstration using honey or know of honey tasting events. Interest and knowledge level of honey in the country is generally low. I believe many people here don't know how honey is actually produced. And teachers in the schools here do not really make any attempt to educate and explain to their kids in details how honey is produced. Many children grow up innocently thinking that honey simply comes from the jars or bottles in the supermarkets or grocery stores.

I often wonder how many people here know about the goodness of honey, its relevance to good health immunity system, or are aware how it can be incorporated into their diet or cooking. The average household knows honey costs much more than table sugar but has no clue how much more extra value they could gain if they and their families eat honey instead of table sugar. Perhaps at most some youngsters will consider grabbing a honey stick from the store to enjoy it but are not bothered by its nutritional content.

Also, as it seems, people here don't really know what honey to look for and what would be considered as good quality honey. They are only familiar with the mass produced honey on supermarket shelves, a homogenous blend that makes each jar have the same mainstream flavour. Many don't know that there is so much more to honey, that honey from each bee colony is really a snapshot of that landscape, the flowers and crop that flourish there, and that time period. They are not aware of how much they are missing out there when it comes to honey and its varying flavour, profiles and facades. Attitudes towards light and dark honey are probably like decades ago where people saw all wine as basically either red or white.

Clueless about the different floral varieties of honey, many people I know have no idea how honey can be ingeniously and creatively used in cooking. Here, the sweet liquid is used mostly in marinating barbeque meats and mixing with water to make throat-soothing or thirst quenching icy honey drink, a popular drink in our hot climate that is supposed to reduce "heatiness in the body". Occasionally, it's also eaten as a sauce for breakfast pancakes and added as a sweetener to herbal teas and fruit juices. However, applying honey on toast or bread like is somewhat strange and bizarre for most locals. And how honey can be spooned and eaten straight from the jar, drizzled over fruit, pancakes, and waffles, or how honey can be used as a natural sweetener in place of sugar in hot drinks and desserts such as puddings are all not common knowledge and practices here.

Easy "Ready-to-Go" Honey Recipes

If you have always found cooking a chore and there's simply no time for it, these ready-to-go honey recipes, some of my most favourites, would definitely suit you. Not only are they easy to prepare, they are also healthy, with honey 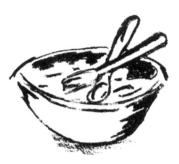 added as a sweetener. Try them! (You can also find these in my free e-book, "Sweet and Sour Recipes - Summer Honey Delights" in my website: http://www.benefits-of-honey.com/sweet-and-sour-recipe.html.)

Fickle Pickly Feat

A zesty, mouth-watering pickled dish that goes perfect with a bowl of plain porridge or simply as a tantalising treat with afternoon tea. Apple cider vinegar makes this dish healthier than ever!

Mix all the ingredients together:

1. Pineapple (1 quarter, skin removed, cut into thin strips)
2. Cucumber (1 quarter, washed, cut into thin strips)

3. White Radish (1 quarter, cut into thin strips)
4. Carrot (1 third, cut into thin strips)
5. Cabbage (3 whole leaves, washed, cut into thin strips)
6. Roasted sesame (1-2 tablespoons)
7. Roasted peanuts (crushed 1-2 tablespoons)
8. Apple cider vinegar (3-4 tablespoons)
9. Honey (3-4 tablespoons)
10. Salt (1 teaspoon)
11. Red chillies (1-2, washed, cut into thin strips)

Store in an air-tight container and chill overnight. Serves 2

Fairies of the Dew Valley

A refreshing bowl of freshly cut honeydew and pineapple resting in a heart-thumping fusion of sweet and citrus bits of dried fruits. A must-try appetizer especially for kicking off a round of barbecued foods. Mixing up the dried fruit bits with succulent fruits certainly does stir up and invigorate the taste buds!

Mix all the ingredients together:

1. Chilled honeydew (1 quarter, cut into small cubes, about 2 by 2 cm)
2. Chilled pineapple (1 quarter, cut into small cubes, about 1 by 1 cm)
3. 5 water chestnuts (remove skin, cut into tiny cubes)
4. 4 dried apricots (cut into tiny cubes)
5. 3 pieces of dried mango (cut into tiny cubes)
6. 2 tablespoons of dried cranberries (cut into tiny cubes)
7. Lime juice (extracted from 4 limes)
8. Cinnamon (a dash, optional)
9. Salt (half teaspoon)
10. 2 tablespoons of honey

Serves 2

Tango Mango Swank

Bring this tangy limed mango-papaya pickle on to satisfy all the pickle lovers! The nutty and spicy kick and pineapple flavour are a perfect match.

Mix all the ingredients together:

1. 1 chilled green mango (remove skin, cut into thin long strips)
2. 1 slice of chilled green papaya (amount equal to that of mango, remove skin, cut into thin long strips)
3. Salt (2 teaspoons)
4. Honey (3-4 tablespoons)
5. Lime juice (extracted from 5 limes)
6. 2 red chillies (washed, cut into thin long strips)
7. Garnish with :
8. A few fresh basil leaves
9. Roasted peanuts (2 tablespoons, coarsely crushed)
10. Walnuts (3 tablespoons, coarsely crushed)

Serves 3-4

Happy Apple Crunch

A jumble of apples and strawberries with a dulcet yoghurt base. With the aromatic yoghurt and pistachio sauce, apples never taste so good!

Mix all ingredients together:

1. 1 chilled green apple (optional skin, washed, cut into small thin slices)
2. 1 chilled red apple (optional skin, washed, cut into small thin slices)
3. 4 dried apricots (cut into tiny bits)
4. 5 chilled strawberries (washed, cut into small thin slices)
5. Lime juice (1 tablespoon)
6. Salt (1 teaspoon)
7. Honey (2 teaspoons)
8. Sprinkle with pistachio nuts (3 tablespoons, remove shell and crush coarsely) just before serving

Serves 2-3

30 Questions with Answers

1.
Question: My hair is dry and dull. Can honey help?

Answer: Massage into the scalp and hair honey with egg yolk. Leave for a 1/2 hour, then wash.

2.
Question: What is Queen Bee's honey and what is its benefit?

Answer: The name for queen bee's honey is "Royal Jelly". It's a very special food made just for the queen bee. (Note: Queen Bee's honey doesn't mean honey produced by the queen bee. The queen bee's job is not to produce honey.)

3.
Question: Does it make a difference if I use Manuka honey or Acacia honey for the Hibernation Diet?

Answer: The floral variety doesn't matter, but 100% pure, unadulterated honey does.

4.

Question: I bought a jar of fresh honey with the comb inside with the honey. Is eating the actual honey comb inside a jar of honey good for you?

Answer: The biggest advantage of eating honey with the comb is -- you can be 100% sure you are eating unprocessed, raw honey that will give you the most health benefits because of all the live enzymes. The wax does not taste fantastic but some people like to chew it like a gum and eat it as roughage to improve bowel system.

5.

Question: How many grams of sugar does honey contain? I have yet to come to a site that gives that information.

Answer: Honey is basically a type of sugar (80%), so if you consume 20g of honey, you are in principle eating about 20g of sugar. The difference between honey and other sugars is that the former is natural and produced by the bees.

6.

Question: How exactly do you use honey to cure infection of yeast or thrush with honey?

Answer: It is an external application treatment, i.e. applying onto the affected area. Many websites advise the following: "Sit on the toilet and apply honey liberally over the affected area. Douche, let it stay for five to ten minutes and then bathe to clean up. Do this twice a day, morning and just before going to bed at night."

7.
Question: I heard that pure honey could be used as a remedy to cuts and scrapes, and it works better than Neosporin. Is it true?

Answer: Indeed honey has been hailed by many as an effective antiseptic for cuts and scrapes. As a natural first aid cure, it absorbs moisture from the air and promotes healing. And its antibacterial properties prevent infection and act as an anti-inflammatory agent. UMF Manuka is a popular honey varietal for wound application due to its strong antibacterial property. Clean the wound and apply raw honey directly.

8.
Question: My daughter has very bad eczema. I was told that honey and cinnamon would help. How does it work?

Answer: Honey and cinnamon have been used as folk remedy for eczema due to their anti-bacterial properties. Honey generally is good for keeping the skin hydrated and there are floral varieties with stronger anti-microbial effects that are popularly used for skin problems, for instance, Manuka UMF honey with its antibacterial potency is used on its own to heal eczema and other skin infections. Hence, naturally, Manuka honey is commonly used with cinnamon for healing the skin.

9.

Question: I have found an unopened plastic jar of honey in the cabinet which I assume has been there quite a while. Is there a reason not to use this old jar of honey?

Answer: In principle, honey does not spoil. But storage conditions are important considerations, e.g. air tight jar to prevent absorption of any moisture, cool temperature, kept away from the sun. All these would affect the quality of the honey - aroma, colour, and taste. A lot of commercial honey uses plastic for bottling due to cost, and plastic is not always the most ideal material for storing food over time (glass is a much better choice for keeping any food as it does not react with food easily.)

If you are not sure how old that jar of honey is, use your discretion, open up, sniff it to see if the smell tells you something, and taste a bit of the honey to decide if you want to further use it.

10.

Question: You say honey doesn't go bad, but my honey has an expiration date. Why is this?

Answer: Liquid honey tends to crystallise over time, making it look lumpy and unappealing on the shelf (though quality is not affected). Thus, for commercial reasons, an expiry date is stated on the honey.

11.

Question: How does the strength of honey compare with that of Karo syrup? How would I substitute honey for Karo syrup?

Answer: A big part of Karo syrup is made of high fructose corn syrup which is a highly processed sweetener. Any unprocessed sweetener like natural honey will always be more beneficial for our body. Honey is about just as sweet as Karo syrup, you can substitute it on an 1-to-1 ratio.

12.

Question: Some types of honey are very smooth, and others seem to clump a lot faster. Does crystallisation affect honey?

Answer: Crystallisation doesn't change the quality of the honey.

13.

Question: I would like to heat up my crystallised honey, but how should I heat it up until it is pourable?

Answer: You can place the crystallised honey in a glass container over hot water to restore the state of the honey. However, never heat honey above 60 degree C. as this will affect the honey's aroma and flavour and destroy its food value, enzymes.

13.

Question: I notice that some of the honey is darker than others, some as dark as molasses. What does this mean?

Answer: Honey varies in colour depending on its varieties; hence whether it's darker or lighter may not be an indicator of its quality. Crystallisation also lightens the colour of honey.

14

Question: Can honey be frozen until you are ready to use it?

Answer: It is fine to freeze honey which you will not be using for months, without harming it. To avoid the hassle of defrosting, I would recommend storing honey in an air tight container in dry, cool place.

15.

Question: I have Seborrhoea Dermatitis on the face and behind the ears. I have read that honey can help. Do you have any ideas?

Answer: Try raw Manuka UMF Honey, which has been reported to be effective in treating Seborrhoea Dermatitis because of its high antibiotic activity.

16.

Question: How can I use honey to treat facial pigmentation problems?

Answer: You may want to try the pumpkin honey face mask, a DIY folk remedy which some people find it effective for treating problems such as freckles and pigmentation.

Instruction: Mix 2-3 table spoons of mashed boiled pumpkin, 1 egg yolk and a teaspoon of honey. Apply on warm face for 10-15 minutes and wash off with cool water. Before putting mask on the face it is necessary to put a hot (not scorching hot) towel for 2-3 minutes.

17.

Question: I am looking for "unpasteurized" on the label when I buy honey. However, is all unpasteurized honey required to be labelled as such? I see many honey products, claiming to be "natural". Can I to assume that all honey with no distinct label is pasteurized?

Answer: "Natural honey" is not equated with "unpasteurized"/"raw". "Natural honey" could mean unadulterated honey, i.e. pure, not added with cane sugar, malt, or glucose. Usually, indeed when honey is not labelled "unpasteurized", it is pasteurized, and nowadays most commercial honey is pasteurized (as opposed to honey you get from the local honey farm).

As for the "pasteurized" labelling, every country has their own set of regulations and requirements. For some countries, the term "unpasteurized" label on honey is prohibited, and you can find the label "raw" instead. Unpasteurized honey is now mostly directly purchased from the local honey farms, which do not exist in places within easy reach for some people.

18.

Question: How do I weigh honey accurately without any mess?

Answer: To measure accurately liquid honey, you can first brush or rub a very thin layer of cooking oil on the inner walls of the measuring cup to prevent the honey from sticking to the cup. (Nowadays, there are also non-stick sprays in the market to replace the need to smear cooking oil onto surfaces.)

19.

Question: What are the benefits of using the honey produced in your own area?

Answer: It is a popular belief that consuming honey produced in your own area could counteract and treat pollen allergies. Some people have reported taking local honey a little bit on a daily basis for several months before the pollen season has made them become tolerant of the allergies.

20.

Question: Do you get the same benefits from raw honey if you put it in coffee or tea (thus heating it)? How is this compared to the heat used in the pasteurization of regular honey?

Answer: To preserve the full goodness of honey, avoid adding piping hot water, as this would not only reduce the aroma and flavour of the honey, but also destroy the natural enzymes present in honey. It's advised that honey be added only when the tea or coffee has cooled down to some extent (not more than 60 °C).

Most commercial honey is pasteurised (even if it's labelled "raw honey"). Honey suppliers have commercial pasteurizing equipments that heat honey quickly to about 70 degrees C for a few minutes and then cool it very quickly. This process will reduce the food value of honey to some extent.

21.
Question: Can I take honey with an empty stomach?

Answer: It's fine to take honey water with an empty stomach. Honey is gentle on the stomach and contains a mix of natural sugars such fructose. Many people take it as a first food in the morning and many athletes take it as an energy booster drink.

22.
Question: Is cactus honey powder made from cactus flower honey? What is special about cactus honey?

Answer: "Cactus honey", marketed as a sugar replacement, is made from the juice of a Mexico-native cactus plant called Agave. It doesn't come from the bees. The name "honey powder" is misleading.

As for what is sold in the market as "honey powder" for baking and cooking purposes, maltodextrin made from corn flour is added to obtain the product in powder form. Honey that has been spray-dried into a fine powder may constitute only a small percentage of the final "honey powder" product.

23.
Question: Can you tell me about honey and milk use for needed childhood weight gain?

Answer: Honey when added to milk has been known to be helpful in improving the digestive system and appetite of children (above 18 months). The fermentable carbohydrates in honey including a variety of oligosaccharides can function as prebiotics and enhance the growth, activity and viability of bifidobacteria in milk, and fermented dairy products such as yoghurts. When children eat well, you don't have to worry about their weight. If they don't like honey in their milk, a spoonful of honey can also be taken directly before bedtime.

24.
Question: I was wondering why and how drinking the boiled cinnamon with honey added can help you burn fat. How is this possible?

Answer: Notice that the combination of honey and cinnamon is a folk remedy, which is not prescribed by medical doctors. Nevertheless, researchers and scientists have claimed that cinnamon's water soluble components, called proanthocyanidins, which are the active ingredients affecting blood glucose, LDL cholesterol, and triglyceride levels. Hence, this spice has been used by many people who have high cholesterol, or are overweight or diabetic.

As for why honey is combined with cinnamon by ancient people, I believe is for a few reasons -- metabolizing of undesirable cholesterol and fatty acid, providing a fuelling mechanism for the body, keeping blood sugar levels balanced and letting your recovery hormones get on with burning fat stores, and making the remedy more palatable (which may not be an important or relevant factor for everyone).

25.

Question: I have a bottle of honey that looks cloudy. Is there any problem with its quality compared to clear honey?

Answer: Cloudiness in honey is due to the presence of pollen, or particles such as wax, flecks of bee pollen, and even bee fragments, which could be in a way everyone would consider as undesirable. Usually, raw honey that is unprocessed or unheated tends to be cloudier than clear honey that is well-filtered and processed. 100%, unprocessed raw honey is more nutritious than processed ones. Commercial honey has been heated and thoroughly filtered so that it looks cleaner and more appealing on the shelf; however its vitamins and minerals are partially destroyed during heating.

26.

Question: I heard that honey could be used as a remedy to minor cuts and scrapes, and it works better than something like Neosporin. Is it true?

Answer: Indeed honey has been hailed by some as an effective antiseptic for cuts and scrapes. Clean the wound and apply raw honey directly.

27.

Question: Can honey help in overcoming the embarrassing issue of bad breath?

Answer: Honey home remedy for bad breath works by reducing the amount of bacteria in the mouth. Try this: Mix 1 teaspoon of Manuka honey , 1/8 teaspoon of cinnamon powder, 1/2 cup hot water and use as a gargle in the morning and evening.

28.

Question: Do you have any tips on how I can deal with my sinus problems using honey?

Answer: Daily, take a tablespoon of honey before bedtime to reduce the occurrence sinus symptoms. It was reported that Ottawa University doctors had found in tests that ordinary honey killed bacteria that caused sinus infections, and did it better in most cases than antibiotics.

29.

Question: How do you apply honey to treat athlete feet?

Answer: This involves rubbing of raw honey on the infected areas before bedtime and leaving it to dry overnight. Cover the treated foot with an old sock. In the morning, wash with water and dry thoroughly.

30.

Question: I have been taking medication for asthma for a long time and would like now to give natural treatment a try. Any advice?

Answer: Honey and cinnamon is a well-known home remedy for asthmatic symptoms. Mix one teaspoon of honey with half teaspoon of cinnamon powder and take the concoction just before going to sleep at night and first thing in the morning. It is not meant to be a rescue or quick-relief medication, but with repeated dosage, many have found to be an effective asthma treatment.

About the Author

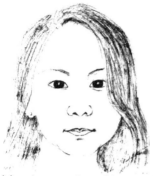

Residing in a country where there is not a single honeybee farm or a trace of beekeeping activity, Ruth Tan speaks from her wealth of personal experience in using honey – how it can detoxify and heal burns, cough, throat inflammation, adrenal fatigue, and infections. Mind-blowing stories of how others have also been healed by the golden liquid fascinate her to record her thoughts about honey in this book.

Ruth Tan is the founder of the popular website Benefits of Honey which is an immensely rich, quality resource on honey and its benefits, and a plethora of health-related issues. Growing everyday with more and more people from all over the world sharing with her health benefits of honey through the website is her conviction that honey is able to make a remarkable difference in the health of this generation and the generations to come.

She is also the author of the Book "Darling, Honey is Good for You!" which introduces honey to young children, telling them what this golden liquid is, where it comes from, and the goodness it brings in a simple language they can appreciate.

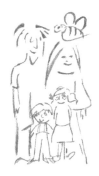

Eating for health has never been sweeter

Discover the amazing health benefits and all the positive spin-offs super-food honey can bring to your life and the lives of your loved ones at
http://www.benefits-of-honey.com

CPSIA information can be obtained
at www.ICGtesting.com
Printed in the USA
LVHW081306101118
596669LV00021B/546/P